Preface

I have lived most of my life under good circumstances. I was born with a roof over my head, I always had food on the table, and my parents are still happily married. Which is more than most can say at this point. However, much of my younger life was spent not knowing that I was dealing with something that has become all to common among those living today. I have severe, chronic depression. There is no cure, and the only help medicine has to offer is in the form of a small pill I take every day to keep me from slipping into a dark funk that will result in my killing myself.

This story is all too common today. I live it, and so many others live it too. However, recently I discovered something that has made a huge difference in my life. I discovered a way to shake off the depression and feel fulfilled in my life. That way I have come to call it the Theory of Connection, and I wish to share it with you in this book.

Some years ago I was on a journey of self-discovery. I had a lot of time to think to myself as I lived in Finland, which is considered to be the happiest country in the world. In my self-reflection I discovered some things, which I have called my pillars. These pillars are what make up me, the foundations upon which my identity, my sense of self, reside.

I am writing this book to teach what I have learned, and so this is written in the sense of a series of thoughts, a collection of memories if you will. I hope that the content you find within will help you in your own journey of self-discovery, and maybe help you to see the world in a different light. If this book has helped you, I urge you to share it with a friend so that they can learn from it as well.

Many of the names have been changed due to privacy, but the stories remain true.

The Theory of Connection

All around us today, people are living alone. During my time in Finland, one of the tasks that was set for me was to speak to as many people as possible each day. As days went on I found that I had begun to tell that there was a certain look, a certain manner of walking that was different from the rest of everyone whom I spoke with.

I soon discovered that there were people in this country who had not spoken in over a year. They lived alone, worked from their homes, and even when out, they kept their heads down and eyed others warily. The more I saw of these people, the more I spoke with them, the more I realized just how out of touch they were with reality. These people lived in fear, uncertain of what was going to happen to them next.

Many of them were completely terrified as I spoke to them in my broken Finnish, and most of them were not happy.

On occasion though, I would say just the right thing, and a stream of Finnish words would flow out of them far faster than my meager experience would allow me to translate, but from reading expressions and body language I could understand the sheer joy they felt from having someone who was brave enough to ask them how their day went. I could have conversations with these people with my limited vocabulary by simply understanding the subject we were on and letting them do all of the talking. They were desperate for a chance to talk to someone, and didn't even know it. When our conversations would inevitably end, many walked away with a smile on their face and a spring in their step that was nowhere to be seen before.

My time in Finland taught me that we all need to have a chance to interact with others. A chance to Connect with them, and share a moment of mutual appreciation for each other. Later on in this book, I will be talking about the effects that this connection has on us, but for now we have a few other things to discuss.

Having lived with this depression my entire life, I saw something in many of the Finns that was all too familiar. A smile that never reached their eyes, a deep longing for someone to listen, and a stature of trying to stay invisible. It reminded me of something I had convinced myself of, 'That I was happier alone.'

This thought was nearly constant in my mind. I had told myself it growing up so many times that it had become almost a mantra, a foundation of who I was. I believed it. I had to. If I didn't I couldn't be myself, because I was only happy when I was alone. The mentalities that created this were the result of my childhood, mistakes and misunderstanding that were not the fault of anyone, because nobody could see into my mind and understand where I went wrong.

Depression

In my early years I was that bookish nerd who was bullied. Sound familiar? I was the kid everyone hated in school because I was always asking the teacher questions, was way too advanced for my class, all of it. I had this passion for learning because it felt so good to have something new to think about. However, slowly, over the course of years, that passion died. I hated school. I hated being with my peers because no matter what I would do, or who I tried to be, I was not accepted, and it hurt. So, I told myself a lie. I was happier alone. I isolated myself and spent time playing video games and reading books. I lazed about in bed as much as I could because I hated the time I spent awake. Eventually, after years of this, I found myself numb.

The human mind is an amazing thing. When dealt with a situation it does

not know how to deal with, it will try hundreds, thousands of possibilities to figure the situation out. We are programmed to learn, designed to interact with the world and find ways to do stuff. However, the mind is also very fragile. If left alone, it will force itself to adapt to short interactions with others. The less time we spend with people, the more desperate we become in our conversations. We try to fit as much as we can into as short of a time as we can. We do all we can to make sure that what conversation we need comes across, sacrificing clarity and simplicity in order to pack the information very compactly. However, the mind is also tough in that it will shut down those sensations that make us feel as though we are not of value. Being in pain is not fun, and our brains don't want us to not be having fun, so we slip into a state of not caring, defending ourselves by shutting down.
    This state is depression. It is a

coping mechanism to deal with rejection, to deal with being alone. Depression is a literal slowing of neural activity. The body conserves energy and uses less throughout the day. I am no evolutionary biologist, but I would venture to guess that it is a mechanism to help an individual return to their tribe should they end up separated.

Which brings us back to these Finnish people I was speaking with. Many of them lived with depression every day. As I came to this understanding, my heart broke for them. I understood what they felt, and began to understand what was going on inside of myself.

I had this need to speak with others. I had this need to spend time conversing, sharing, learning, becoming, socializing. It was an instinctual need on the same level as hunger. We all have this need, and we all need to act on it.

There are many studies out today which point to the necessity of human contact. A prime example is found in the worst punishment we as humans have ever come up with, isolating someone. Solitary Isolation is a punishment used in prison for the worst of the worst. The effects of being alone for too long are known to be the cause of the individual to go insane, to lose control of themselves and become something closer to a beast than a person.

Ugly Truth

When a child is born, if they receive no physical contact their likelihood of living is decreased dramatically. Without touch, an infant will die. This goes to show the sheer need we as humans have to not only be around others and speak with them, but also have physical touch and contact.

Yet, many of our parents or grandparents live alone. They spend their days with nobody to speak to, and many of them also end up depressed. In Western Society today, it is considered a rite of passage to move out of one's parents' house. Getting out and living on your own is so emphasized that many parents do not even give their children a choice, but kick them out of their home the day they turn 18. The second their child becomes an adult, I have seen so many families cut their connection with each other, and then complain that they never see one another.

Because of this mentality, many parents push their children to be adults only when they reach the age of 18. Before hitting this magical, imaginary line, the child is expected to behave like, and be treated like, a child. No parent honestly knows what they are doing as they raise a child, and the transition from child to adult is never given a chance to happen because of parents not allowing children to learn how to be independent.

Through growing up there is a concept that everything should go right for you, that if something happens, it isn't your fault. Everyone goes through it. You believe yourselves to be entitled to a world rolling over for you. That the world should be safe, fair, and kind. These thoughts and behaviors, in a healthy development, would have been removed between the ages of 13 and 16, as a child learns self-accountability and work ethic. Instead this mentality continues and doesn't resolve until the ages of 20 to 30.

However, they are not taught. As such we have a group of people who do not see the world as it really is, and try to change something that isn't real to suit their fancy. One cannot make positive changes to anything unless they fully understand what they are attempting to do.

As the parents push against the mentality that they cultivated, it causes the children to become disenchanted with their parents. It is hard having someone around who will not listen to you, does not see you for yourself, and is always getting on your case for things that may or may not be in your control. Because of this, as a child ages they drift away from their parents, and cut ties down to a minimum.

With their ties cut, the parents find themselves aging alone. Left with a marriage if they are lucky, if only for a few years. In the time where society would have them preparing to enter retirement, and enjoy the golden years of their life, they find themselves suffering from all sorts of health problems due to the infirmity of age. They have lived their life and lost their chance to enjoy it, and all that is left is another broken family, and the elderly die alone.

This scenario is a little extreme compared to what will happen in many cases, but the point I am making is this - Nobody is to blame for this. It is simply a natural flow of events that will take place, should certain factors line up. It does not have to be this way. In my own family, we are fairly close. Do I visit my parents as often as I should? Probably not, but it is something I am working on. All of this is a process. One does not build Rome in a day.

Communication

Many families I know have confided in me as individuals that they all want to be closer to one another, but for most of them it ends up being the same situation - They do not know how to talk to one another in a way that will allow them to understand each other. We want to understand, but cannot get past the barriers that bar our way to having a peaceful conversation filled with understanding. Often the reasons for this lie in events of our past, barely remembered rules that we are forcing ourselves to live by, consciously or unconsciously.

What does any of this have to do with overcoming depression? The family unit is, or should be, our closest network of individuals we can rely on for help in hard times. We have the need, the primal urge to have a family, a place where we belong. This is the reason that many kids in broken homes end up joining gangs, a topic which could fill its own book. Depression is directly associated with isolation, and so it is of key importance to ensure that you are not alone.

In order not to be alone though, we need to be able to communicate. It is scary, I know. I am one of the most introverted people I know of, preferring to spend my days in my office typing away at my computer. However, it is of utmost importance. Just like the Finns who had not spoken to another soul in a year, we can end up broken and depressed, not even aware of what or why.

There are a lot of forms of communication. Talking about the way we talk is its own field of study, so I will suffice it to say that the main methods we use are speaking and touch. With our words we can express complex concepts, share them with others even through time by writing them down.

Through touch we can say things that words cannot describe, we can show our pain, we can give comfort.

However, speaking is not the same as communicating. Holding someone in your arms does not tell them why you are hurting. Communication has a very important suffix. Co- means joint, mutual, or common. It means together. To communicate requires the conversation to go both ways. If one is speaking, and the other is not listening, the words have no meaning. Just as we must speak, we must listen, and we must listen with an open mind and an open heart. If we enter a conversation with our predefined opinion of someone, how can we get to know who they really are? People change over time, yesterday's enemy can become today's friend.

Now, to get deeper into the hows of communication, let's lay some groundwork. Each of us have a series of 'pillars' in us. These pillars are things we can communicate about, they are things such as an appreciation for art, a favorite pet, an understanding of algebra, etc. We all have many of these pillars, and in order to communicate with each other we have to have some common ground between the pillars.

Just having a common pillar is not all that it takes though. You see, each of us has a different size and shape to our pillars. This is because of our individual experiences and understandings. Each of our perspectives are different, because of the small differences in our pillars. These differences are what lead to difficulty in communicating.

When we have differences in our pillars, the way we see our pillars is also different. When describing it, there will be points and features that each of us disagree on, but for the most part if our understanding is sound, we will have similarities in our pillars. These are the points which we can communicate on in order to help build relationships. The pillars are far more complex than just this, and deserve their own book, just like many of these concepts, and so what we care about right now are the details in the pillars, the bits and pieces we can share between each other.

    Sharing these parts of the pillars are how we can bond and begin to overcome the depression that takes over our minds. Think back to the last time you had a good conversation. Something got your mind going, and you ended up talking for a long time about one subject. Were you depressed during that? Even if the subject was a sad one, I highly doubt it. Storytelling requires too much brain function to allow for depression. Did you feel good after it was all over? Did you at least feel better?

The Pillars

Let me tell you the story of Greg (Name changed for privacy). Greg was my mentor when I first started my internship as a machinist. For those who do not know, Machining is a manufacturing method where you cut metal into the shape that it needs to be. It's really precise and really slow. Because of the nature of the exact products I was working on, Jet engine parts, the job was also incredibly stressful.

Back to Greg. Greg was short, squat, and round. He was not exactly fat, but definitely heavier, with a lot of muscle underneath. He was balding, so he kept his head shaved, and had a short red beard. He was practically the stereotype for a machinist: loud, rough, and scary. If you recall my mention earlier, I am not like that. I am small, thin, and built much closer to a skinny hobbit.

The first day I met him was right after he had some dental surgery, so he came to work to greet me and then left for the day. My first impressions of him were bad, to say the least. By the end of the first week I thought him to be lazy, slow, and stupid. He seemed to drag wherever he was going, and would not answer hardly any of my questions.

Beyond all of that, he was an intimidating figure, even though he was an inch shorter than me. (I am 5'4", so he was pretty short) So, as time went on I grew scared of him. I would back into my professional tone with him, and kept myself to myself. I worked hard, learned what I could, and tried not to make any mistakes. He was a good enough teacher, when he was teaching, so I felt like we would be able to get along this way until my training was complete.

As I am going to show you, people are rarely as they seem. I had built a pillar that was Greg, but the pillar was nothing like the real thing. This is why it is so dangerous to judge others based on what we think we see.

Greg was a much better person than I was. He probably knew that I was terrified of him, so not a month into our relationship he worked to crack my shell. He was quite the master at it, each day coming in with a new topic to try his hand at throwing at me. Finally, he hit on the one that would eventually break me open and lead me to an obsession I still have today.

Greg told me about his new garden he was putting in. He talked about how he had borrowed a tractor from his neighbor to till over some land, and the work he was putting in on it. At this time in my life I was beginning to study the concepts of permaculture, a gardening principle. My pillar was still small, and he had experience he could draw from to help me grow my own pillar. Before I knew it I was talking to him about some theories I had, and he was telling me how bad they were. We spent some of our down time discussing it and formed a friendship from there.

As days passed, he would come to me with that day's events in the garden, such as how he had ended up digging up slabs of asphalt that were buried there, meaning he would need to either spend weeks digging them up or move the garden. I would try to help him come to a solution, simply because that was the only way I knew how to have a conversation, and he would listen.

Through him, I became obsessed with gardening. I was still living with my parents, and ended up taking over the family garden, only to fail at it miserably. However, I loved every moment I spent out in the garden, thinking about what I was learning and how I could get the system to work. When I was out in my garden, my depression was gone. I loved and enjoyed being out there, even though I was terrible at it.

As days went by I slowly lost those

thoughts that Greg was lazy, slow, and stupid. I realized that he was so much more than he had seemed on the surface. It did not happen all at once, but eventually I saw Greg as a person, instead of just my mentor.

Greg is a good man. He prefers to be efficient, and spends time thinking how to solve a problem with less work. He doesn't talk with a complex vocabulary, but speaks so that even an idiot can understand him, a skill I wish I could figure out. He was never slow, he just simply took his time to do things right the first time. When faced with an obstacle he would look at it from every angle before proceeding. He was an excellent machinist, and an even better mentor.

From Greg I learned that it is important not to think we know people, because they will prove us wrong. I came to enjoy working with him, and as time went on I found more and more in common between the both of us.

Because he took out the effort to find a common pillar between the two of us, he remains a good friend to this day.

To spend a moment summarizing what I have been saying to this point, the Theory of Connection is that if we connect ourselves with others we may be able to end the depression in our lives. However, there is more to this than just simply connecting with others. We also need to connect with ourselves.

The Shadow

Inside all of us exists something called the Shadow. The Shadow is our darkness, those thoughts telling us to do something horrible, something awful. We all have it. We bury it because those thoughts are dark, and we do not want to see them. This darkness inside of us is a part of us.

Why do we have such a darkness inside of us? Rewinding time back a long time, humans needed those thoughts to keep them safe. The world was just as dark and scary as those thoughts, so being ready to flip in a moment was necessary to our survival. Is the darkness in this Shadow the same darkness of depression? No. Depression is a lack of everything, a missing, gaping hole. This darkness, the Shadow, is material, and a direct opposite to the behaviors we normally allow ourselves to exhibit.

The Shadow is just as much a part of our identity as the rest of us. We can choose to ignore it, but every time we do so, when we are depressed, the thoughts linger in the void, growing, festering. These dark thoughts tell us to do things that we would never do. Things that involve killing ourselves, hurting others, even killing others. Because of our depression, we cannot so easily overcome the thoughts by pushing them away. So, we are going to go on a bit of a side tangent on how to deal with those thoughts.

When dealing with a dark, intrusive thought, I have found that the best manner of attack is to acknowledge it. Think things such as, "I could do that. But then So and so would be sad." Adding a consequence to the dark thoughts helps to quell them. If this doesn't work, a few other techniques are to tell yourself that you don't want to, or a personal favorite - "I don't have the energy to get out of bed today. How would I have the energy to kill myself?"

Now, if you are having recurring suicidal thoughts, especially when you begin to make a plan, I urge you to reach out to someone you love and trust, or to the Suicide Hotline. (1-800-273-8255). While everyone deals with these thoughts, when depressed, the barriers to acting on these things is severely reduced. Even if you can't tell them about what is going on, they are there to just talk to you. There is no shame in calling the hotline, they are there so that you can make a connection, even if the purpose of the connection is to help you get through another day.

Alright, back to the shadow. It is very important that we come to accept the Shadow as a part of us, because it is not going away anytime soon. In order to integrate the Shadow into ourselves, we have to know and understand our fears and our desires. I encourage you to take a few minutes after finishing this section to think about what you are afraid of, what things you want most in life, and who you believe yourself to be.

In order to understand anyone else, we have to first understand ourselves, at least to some basic sense. The pillars that make up our identity are those things we choose to perceive ourselves as. This is why concepts such as the law of attraction work so well. By changing who you believe yourself to be, you are actually changing who you really are.

There is only one you. That is you. But then, who are you? That is a choice you can make each and every day. I am not meaning on the lines of 'today I am a police officer, tomorrow I will perform heart surgery.' I am meaning the personality traits, like your solid work ethic or your love of poetry, they're malleable. Just like with Greg and I, our pillars can shift and change, and eventually we can become something we were not.

Remember, everyone around you is a human too. They each have their own needs, desires, insecurities and flaws. They struggle with self-worth. They try their best. Each and every one of them has their own past, their own experiences, their own pillars.

Atoms

Let's take a moment to dive into the sun for a thought experiment. It's pretty hot in here, eh? If we focus in on a single atom, we can follow it along a fairly linear path. The atom moves forward, forward, forward, until it runs into something. Another atom. Now, only a few things can happen here. One or both of the atoms have to bounce away, or they will fuse together. Let's look at the case where an atom bounces away.

Each of those atoms represent one of us. For the briefest moments we are in contact with another atom, another person, and have a chance to see and interact with them. We do not know the path they took to get to us, though we can have some idea, and we do not know where they will go after we separate. The only one who knows the entirety of our past is us. We will never know the experience of years that any other person has, so the best we can do is give each other the benefit of the doubt.

Why are we talking about me? Well, I don't know anyone better than I know myself. I can't speak for them because I only exist in myself. So, for now I am going to relate my findings from some meditations I did a while back, and then we will see how we can apply them to you.

Before I can get into the Quadrants, first we need to know what the Axis are. There are two Axis, just like on a normal graph. In the case of X and Y, instead we have Creation and Consumption. Now, don't run away just yet. We aren't going to do any math. It helps if you understand geometry for this, but that is only because I used geometry when creating it to help me understand because I'm a huge nerd.

The first Axis, Creation, has two states. Being in the positive, or actively creating, and being in the negative, or passively creating. The second Axis, Consumption, is likewise. Being in the positive here is actively consuming, while in the negative is passively consuming.

So, put them together to make a plus sign, and you have a handy graph that has four quadrants. In the top right is the state of active creation and consumption, while in the bottom left is the state of passive creation and consumption. Top left is active creation with passive consumption, and bottom right is passive creation and active consumption.

Why do these matter? These two axis are what form my own personal foundation based on two of the things I hold highly valuable. Namely, Creating and Consuming. Short side tangent about consuming, people have told me that it is useless to consume content all the time. I disagree. What are you doing right now? Consuming content that I

created, and through it gaining

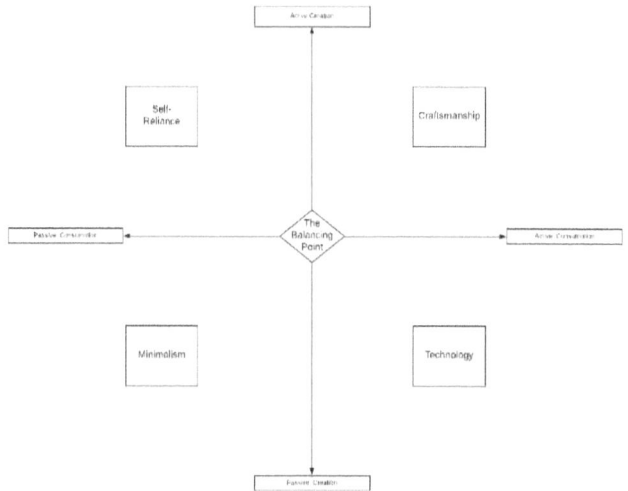

knowledge which will hopefully allow you to create in the future, or at least better yourself.

Now, there is a difference between blind entertainment and consuming information. When we are entertained we gain nothing but the emotional gratification. When we are consuming, we learn deeper and gain real value from the act. Consumption is a necessary part of Connection, because if everyone was a creator, who would consume?

Self-Reliance

And, back to the main topic. Where were we? Ah, right. The Axis. I cannot vouch for others, and it is something that you will need to meditate on yourself, but for me these are the two axis upon which my psyche, my whole identity is built. I have a pillar in each of these quadrants which may be familiar to you.

Starting in the top left, in actively creating and passively consuming, I have the pillar of Self-Reliance. The core concept of this pillar is that my stuff can help other people act. Self-Reliance is a huge topic nowadays, and one that I love to study and contemplate. Even this book was spurred on by the concept of Self-Reliance, because honestly I am hoping to make some income from it while being able to help other people.

Self-Reliance gurus today all talk about the hustle, about creating something with your own two hands, about letting go of everyone around you and becoming the influencer, the king essentially. However, what would happen if we all became Self-Reliant? Many, many bad things would happen, but one of the worst is that we would no longer be standing on the shoulders of those who came before us. To be blindly Self-Reliant is to forget our history, which causes us to repeat it.

What does any of this have to do with depression? My answer is most definitely. You see, when we are too far away from the center of the grid, we start becoming obsessed and blinded by our pillars. Having the pillars is most certainly a good thing, but if we take our self-reliance too far and go live out in the woods to cut ties with everyone in order to be totally self-reliant, what do we gain but misery? The fastest way into depression is to run headfirst towards a single pillar.

There he is! Doom and gloom me

has reared his head! Darkness, Begone! (Kung-fu noises)

Ahem. Now that that is out of the way, let's move on to the next quadrant. We are going to go down to the bottom left, where there is passive creation and consumption. The pillar I have in this quadrant is Minimalism. The reason for this is the understanding that my stuff is not what matters to me.

This might not be the same for you, and that is fine. Everyone is different. However, I have seen that most people who become hardcore minimalists tend to have a similar story of obsession with consumption leading them down a depressing and lonely road. So, they get rid of everything in order to find a place where it isn't the things, but the people who matter to them.

I don't have the same story, honestly I just hate clutter. If I don't need it I don't need it. However, the ideas that these minimalists have has really resonated with me. They all were coming from a place where they had everything and were depressed, and then let go of it and seemingly cured their depression. As I contemplated this idea I found the basis of the Theory of Connection. The reason that all of this works.

The main concept for a Minimalist is the understanding and knowledge that stuff is not connection. This realization brought about an epiphany for me. I had not realized the importance of connection until then. You see, all of this points back to a simple concept. Humans are a tribal species. We live for social contact. We have to have it. If we don't, the result is depression.

Technology

Connection is the opposite of Depression. This, in its most simple form, is the Theory of Connection. Take a moment and contemplate that concept. Connection is the opposite of Depression. When we are connected it is nearly impossible to be depressed. Being connected is such a powerful biological tool that we cannot escape it.

Now, does that mean go out to the club and party to cure depression? Probably not. Depression is a mental illness. Partying doesn't fix things, it usually makes things worse. In my own experience, I have found that most often my worst days are the days that follow having been alone for too long. The days where I don't feel productive and haven't had the chance to create something worthwhile. The times when I have done nothing but binge-watch shows.

Each of those is a positive feedback loop, which is incredibly dangerous. Depression has a habit of telling us that we are better off alone so that we don't hurt anyone around us. As is, I struggle even writing this because I worry that someone is going to be hurt by what I say, but that is just life with depression.

Am I saying to go out and talk to people every time you are depressed? Absolutely not. Some days it is all you can do to just lay on the couch. If you manage that, good job. This is hard. That being said, if you have the energy, talk to someone you love about something you love. Notice what happens after you finish that conversation. Are you still feeling depressed? For me, most of the time I am not. In fact, I, the super introvert, actually feel good after a conversation.

And now, on to the third quadrant. Technology. It is found in the bottom right corner, representing passive creation and active consumption. A simple rule of technology is that an individual does not have the means to produce a smartphone. As is, having a smartphone is necessary in order to do anything nowadays.

Technology represents the collaboration of any individuals for the benefit of one. Not to mention, it is useful. However, it is easy to take things too far with technology. When we start giving up our decisions to the technology, we become enslaved to it. Our time, our attention becomes a means to serve the device. Social Media has a certain skill in taking over our lives and we end up spending hours upon hours consuming content with little to no thought for ourselves.

This is the danger of the pillar of Technology. A danger I struggle with even today. Unfortunately, it is so much easier to just watch one more video, scroll down one more swipe, and leave things for later. However, Technology of itself is not, nor ever will be, evil. Technology is a tool, just like a machete or a shovel. Here in the USA we view machetes as weapons, but we do not generally live in a place where it is used as a tool. In most South American countries it is simply a tool, just like a shovel. People don't look twice.

Technology allows us to reach out and be with other people incredibly easily, should we allow ourselves to use it properly. Machines help our lives become easier and gives us more time to spend doing different tasks. Would you rather use a mortar and pestle to make a smoothie or a blender? I certainly like my blender.

Craftsmanship

By now I hope that you may have noticed somewhat of a pattern in the pillars. Each one has both good and bad associated with it. We can view it from multiple places, depending on where we are at. Let's go back to the chart for a moment.

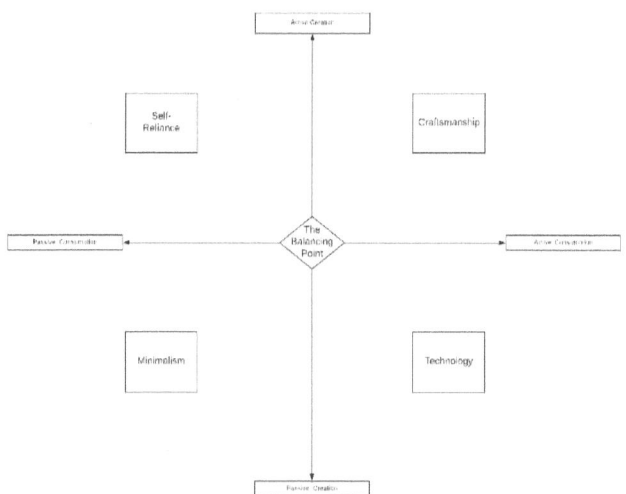

Among all of these pillars is one more thing. Us. We stand somewhere among the pillars and can choose to move about consciously. When we 'put ourselves in someone's shoes', we are walking to where they stand, and viewing the world, the pillars around them, from the way they understand them, from the way they see them.

If applied well, these principles would help each of us understand one another, and many more problems than depression would cease. I invite you to pause for a moment and think about what this book has taught you before we enter the final quadrant. What has resonated with you? What has conflicted with how you view the world?

Now, take another moment to walk around the pillars of life seeking to understand them. Understanding more than just what is visible of the pillars allows us to do so much more.

The final pillar is one that took me a long time to understand. To be honest, I still don't understand it to the fullest. This one, at the crux of both creation and consumption, is Craftsmanship. For the longest time I believed that this was the epitome of existence. This was the be all end all. This was everything. It is not. You see, I was standing far into the distance of active creation and consumption, believing that if we aren't going at full speed all the time and mastering everything we do, we are failures. This is where I was viewing Craftsmanship from the side that prevents connection. The pillar of Craftsmanship had blocked my view of the pillar at the very center of the grid. Connection. We shall talk about that pillar soon.

    I firmly believed that if I didn't spend all of my time working on, or near this pillar, I was not worth it. So, every second spent near the other pillars tortured me, and told me how horrible I was because I couldn't dedicate myself to something I believed to be so simple. This was not the cause of my depression, but a feedback loop that amplified it.

It wasn't until I realized that we are all humans, not robots, that I began this long journey myself. We cannot go at full power all the time. We need rest, we need blank space. Standing next to the pillar of Craftsmanship, everything else was so small in comparison. Once when I finally stepped away, to a more centered location, that I realized what had happened.

There is nothing wrong with Craftsmanship, in fact if used properly it can connect us better than most of the other pillars. The master passes on everything to their apprentice, and this relationship forms the strongest types of bonds, born only from living and working together constantly. Now, those bonds can be both positive and negative, but that is a topic for another day.

The whole history of humanity is one of standing on the shoulders of our ancestors. We honor them by our actions taken from our learning that has been passed on. We connect to them through this pillar.

I have done what this book is trying to tell you not to do. I have stepped too far away from the center, too far away from connection. My understanding and perception of the world was warped because of where I stood. I didn't see things the way they really were, let alone understand them. So, whenever I would try to converse with another, or even be with them, I could not see nor understand them the way they truly were.

Whenever I was with another we would end up viewing the pillars that connected us from different sides, so it was impossible to get along with others. Because of that, my isolation only got worse. It wasn't until I began to move and see the pillars from more sides than one that I realized my mistake.

I used to view other's success as my own failure. Because of that I wanted nothing more than to have everyone else be as miserable as me. It was toxic and dangerous, and brought on by the misunderstanding of what it means to be proud of what we accomplish in craftsmanship.

I thought that I had to feel proud of everything I did, and in order to do so the world had to recognize me. That is not the case. Having pride and feeling accomplished are completely separate. Pride relies on an external source, while feeling accomplished is internal. In finally understanding the truth, I was able to move to where everything matters, and where we can find peace.

The Balancing Point

The final piece to this theory, the culminating purpose and the reason I am sharing it, is this. The Balancing Point. The point where we find ourselves the most connected. The point where we can freely move away from in order to understand another, but can return to in order to clearly understand ourselves.

The Balancing Point, at least for me, lies right in the middle of the graph. Right at the origin. It is centered on everything else, and allows for an understanding of reality without being distorted. When we stand on The Balancing Point we can see the world as it truly is. We understand that we are not bound to a single pillar, but can move about as we need to understand another, and we can finally understand ourselves.

By standing in The Balancing

Point, it becomes easier to speak to anyone. Now, this, in and of itself, is not the cure to depression. If it was something so simple, we would have eliminated the disease by now. No, there is more to it than that. However, this is the first step towards healing from depression.

When we stand on The Balancing Point, and finally view reality through the correct lens, we can begin to break free from the darkness that holds us down. By connecting with others, our depression begins to fade and life becomes somewhat easier. We begin to be capable of working together with others in order to accomplish goals larger than ourselves. We begin to see the ways that everyone's pillars connect, and can start to move in a way that will help us to become free.

Now, how do we apply all of this into simple, actionable tasks? I will say this now, that if I gave the answer to that, you would not listen. There is only so much a book can do for you. However, I am here to point you down the path to begin this yourself.

Take a step back from yourself. Find a quiet spot and a few uninterrupted hours. Review yourself. Make a list of what is most important to you and find what your own pillars are. Once you have done this, embrace the shadow. We all have one, and it tells us so much about who we really are.

Let the emotions all come out. Anger, rage, sadness, joy. Then, when all that is left is you, follow the path that you find. Focus on your connections, and find those around you who you can understand.

www.ingramcontent.com/pod-product-compliance
Lightning Source LLC
Chambersburg PA
CBHW030508220526
45464CB00006B/2702